Irresistibly Yummy Ketogenic Cookbook

57 Keto Diet Recipes For Quicker Weightloss And Healthy Living

DEBBIE CLAWSON

ISBN-13:978-1515263746

ISBN-10:1515263746

DEDICATION

To Rudy and Brian, your presence brings me joy – always!

TABLE OF CONTENTS

INTRODUCTION

Understanding The Keto Diet

A keto diet is a low carbohydrate, high fat and moderate protein diet that causes the body to produce ketones in the liver which are then used as energy.

When a person consumes high or normal carbohydrate, the body produces glucose and insulin which are easily converted and used by the body as energy. Glucose is the preferred or main energy source that is selected over any other source of energy while insulin helps to process the glucose in the bloodstream. Here, fats are not needed but are merely stored.

However, when the carb intake is lowered, the body enters a state of ketosis. During this state, the body produces ketones which are the by-products of the broken down fats in the liver. The body initiates ketosis to help people with low food intake survive.

The main objective of a well-structured keto diet is to force the body into this metabolic state. This is accomplished by starving the body of carbohydrates and not calories. Our bodies adjust easily to what it is given. Once it is devoid of carbohydrate and overloaded with fats, it will start to burn ketosis as its number one energy source for normal day to day functions.

It takes about 2 to 7 days for the body to adjust to this diet and go into ketosis. This is also dependent on the individual's body type, levels of activity and what is being eaten. Exercising on an empty stomach, restricting carbohydrate intake to 20g or less per day and taking lots of water are some of the fastest ways to get into ketosis.

For a normal person starting a ketogenic diet and eating 25-40g of net carbs daily, the total process of adaptation should take about 2 weeks. To attain ketosis within 1 week, cut carbs down to fewer than 15g.

With a ketogenic diet, there will be no need for you to worry about calories as the fats and proteins are filling and will keep you full for an extended period of time. However, if you exercise, you must be more vigilant as exercise comes with a greater calorie deficit that must be replenished.

Be sure to always consult your physician if you have reservations about starting a ketogenic diet. Nevertheless, you MUST see a physician if you come from a family with a history of diabetic or pre-existing conditions because higher intake of protein will definitely put a strain on the kidneys.

Benefits Of A Keto Diet

Besides its obvious weight loss benefit, the ketogenic diet has been widely proven to improve cholesterol, blood sugars, and reduce heart diseases. It is already a well-established form of treatment for epilepsy and research is presently going on to discover ways it can be used to treat other neurological conditions.

It also helps to eliminate irritable bowel syndrome, dementia and Alzheimer as well as to regulate menstruation.

Basically, it operates in a rather different way than medications. While scientists have discovered several different mechanisms of action leading to the diet's success, one significant theme is that instead of causing sedation, one common side-effect of medication, this diet makes the individual more alert and focused.

In a nutshell, a few benefits of the diet are:

Weight Loss - As your body burns fat as the primary energy source, it will start to use the stored fat as an energy source while you are in a fasting state.

Energy - since your body now has better and more dependable energy source, you will begin to feel more energized all through the day. Fats have been confirmed as the best molecule to burn as fuel.

Fighting Hunger - Fat is satiating. You will feel 'fuller' for a longer period of time as a result hunger cravings, common in other forms of dieting, will be almost non-existent.

Blood Sugar -According to documented studies, there is a decrease of LDL cholesterol after a while which eliminates ailments such as type 2 diabetes.

Cholesterol - this diet brings about an improvement in triglyceride levels and cholesterol levels which are most associated with the buildup of arterial.

Eliminating Acne - latest research has shown that it leads to a reduction in skin inflammation and acne lesions within 12 weeks.

What To Eat

Keto dieting requires lots of planning ahead. If you want to get to a ketogenic state quickly, you need to have a workable diet plan.

While 20-30g of net carbohydrate is recommended for daily dieting, you will enter ketosis faster is you restrict your carb intake to less than 15g a day. Strive to keep your glucose level as low as possible and be aware of the net carb of each meal. A net carb is the total dietary carbohydrate without the total fiber.

For example, 1 cup of broccoli contains 6gcarb and 2g fiber. To calculate the net carb, simply take the total carb (6g) and subtract the dietary fiber (2g). This will leave us with a net carb of 4g.

The ideal percentage of keto consumption is 5% carbohydrate, 70% fats and 25% protein. Your carbohydrates should mostly come from vegetables, dairy and nuts. Do not eat refined carbohydrates like wheat (pastas, cereals, breads,), starch (legumes, beans, potatoes) or fruit.

The best choice of vegetables is always dark green and leafy. Your meals should mostly be a protein with vegetables, and an extra side of fat. Examples of these are chicken breast in olive oil, with cheese and broccoli; Steak topped with butter, and a spinach side sautéed in olive oil.

If you find yourself hungry throughout the day, snack on peanut butter, seeds, nuts and cheeses to curb your appetite.

The diet's main sources of fat include:

- Butter
- Heavy cream

- Oils (coconut, vegetable, olive, etc.)

Many stricter forms of the diet do not allow the following foods:

- Pasta
- Potatoes
- Rice
- Candy
- Bread
- Cereals

The most common low-carb vegetables include:

Vegetable	Amount	Net Carbs
Lettuce (Romaine)	1/2 Cup	0.2
Spinach (Raw)	1/2 Cup	0.1
Cauliflower (Steamed)	1/2 Cup	0.9
Cauliflower (Raw)	1/2 Cup	1.4
Bok Choi	1/2 Cup	0.2
Broccoli (Florets)	1/2 Cup	0.8
Cabbage (Green Raw)	1/2 Cup	1.1
Kale steamed	1/2 Cup	2.1
Collard Greens	1/2 Cup	2
Green Beans steamed	1/2 Cup	2.9

At the start of the keto diet plan, you may still have intense sugar cravings as most people do but this will dissipate within a couple of weeks.

Sweeteners can be of help during this period. However, you must be careful because even things that are listed 'carb-free' may still contain carbs. Also, to not forget to take into consideration the net carbs of the sweetener when writing your keto diet plan.

Recommended Sweeteners Include:

Sucralose or splenda - which is usually sold in granulated form. It contains bulking agents which reduces the sweetness. One packet of splenda contains1 net carb.

Stevia - Also known as the sweet leaf, stevia is a natural herb that is gotten by extracting the sweetener inside the leaf as a sugar substitute. It has no vitamins, minerals or calories. It is extremely sweet, about 200 times sweeter than sugar so use sparingly. It can be bought in liquid forms or granulated forms.

Erythritol - A sugar alcohol naturally found in vegetable and fruits. It contains about 70% sugar sweetness so you may need to add a little more than normal. It should also be safely consumed at a maximum of 1 gram per kilogram of body weight.

Xylitol causes tooth decay, according to research so do not use. Steer clear of Aspartame as well.

Changes In The Body

Your body is accustomed to the straightforward routine of breaking carbohydrates down and using them as energy. To accomplish this process, it has built up a resource of enzymes overtime and has only a handful of enzymes for handling fats. As a result, the body merely stores them.

Now, your body has to handle the increase in fats and the lack of glucose. To do this, it has to build up new enzyme supplies. Once your body is induced to a ketogenic state, it will use up the left over glucose it can find, then switch over to the glycogen in the muscles. This may lead to lack of energy and other minor ailments in the first week such as:

- Headaches
- Dizziness
- Mental fogginess
- Aggravation
- Flu-like symptoms colloquially known as the Keto-Flu

These symptoms are normal and will disappear after a week. It is simply due to your electrolytes being flushed out since the ketosis has a diuretic effect. Ensure you drink lots of water and increase your sodium intake. This will help to replenish the electrolyte and help with water retention as well.

Once the body becomes adapted to keto, it will then be able to fully use the fats as its main source of energy. Athletes on this diet do not need to be afraid of a drop in performance after the first week.

KETO BREAKFAST RECIPES

Enjoy these low carb muffins especially on a cold morning. These moist and fully satisfying muffins are pleasantly tasty with a spread of butter.

Lemon Blueberry Muffins
Yields: 15 muffins

<u>Ingredients</u>

2 eggs

1 cup heavy cream

4 ounces fresh blueberries

2 cups Almond Flour

½ tsp. baking soda

1/8 cup melted butter

½ tsp flavoring or lemon extract

5 packets splenda, stevia or any other artificial sweetener

½ tsp dried lemon zest

¼ tsp. salt

<u>Directions:</u>

1. Preheat oven to 350 Fahrenheit degrees. Place the cupcake papers in separate muffin holes of standard sized 12 count muffin pan.

2. Combine cream and almond flour. Add eggs one after the other, and stir until it is well mixed.

3. Add sweetener, butter, flavoring, spices, baking soda and mix.

4. Add blueberries and mix until it is evenly distributed.

5. Next, spoon the mixture into pan, ensuring each cupcake paper is about 1/2 full.

6. Bake until golden or for about 20 minutes. Leave it to cool. Serve with butter.

Nutritional Information per muffin:

Calories 184, protein 5 g, fat17 g, carb 6 g, fiber 2 g.

Tasty Cheese Muffins

Ingredients

2 eggs

½ tsp. baking soda

1/8 cup melted butter

2 cups Almond Flour

½ tsp dried thyme

1 cup of sour cream

½ cup shredded Muenster

1 cup shredded cheddar or Colby jack

¼ tsp. salt

Directions:

1. Preheat oven to 400F degrees. Place the cupcake papers in separate muffin holes of standard sized 12 count muffin pan.

2. Combine the dry ingredients and almond flour.

3. Get a separate bowl, break and beat the eggs lightly in it and then add sour cream and butter and mix.

4. Add the liquid mixture to the mixture of almond flour. If it seems too thick, add 1 tablespoon of heavy cream or water.

5. Add cheese and mix together until it is evenly distributed.

6. Spoon mixture into muffin pans, ensuring each is about 3/4 full.

7. Bake for 5 minutes at 400 degrees.

8. Turn down the oven temp to 350 then bake for another 20- 25 minutes or until golden. Leave it to cool. Serve with butter.

Nutritional Information

 Per muffin: total of 2 net grams

Calories 166, fat15 g, protein 6 g, carb5 g, fiber 3g

Sour Cream Blueberry Muffins
Yields: 15 muffins

Ingredients

2 cups almond flour

½ tsp. baking soda

2 eggs

1/4 cup erythritol

1 cup sour cream

1/8 cup melted butter

4 ounces fresh blueberries

½ tsp. salt

Directions

1. Preheat oven to 350degrees. Place the cupcake papers in separate muffin holes of standard sized 12 count muffin pan.

2. Combine the dry ingredients and almond flour.

3. Get a separate bowl, break and beat the eggs lightly in it and then add sour cream and butter and mix until smooth.

4. Combine the sour cream mixture and almond flour mixture, stirring until well mixed.

5. Add blueberries and mix until it is evenly distributed.

6. Spoon the mixture into muffin cups, ensuring each is about 1/2 full.

7. Bake until golden or for about 20 minutes. Leave to cool. Serve with butter.

Nutritional Information

Per muffin: total of 3 net grams

Calories: 147, protein 5g, fat13g, carb 5g, fiber 2g .

Sugary Cinnamon Donut Muffins
Yield: 12

<u>Ingredients</u>

For the Donut Muffins:

2 large Eggs

½ cup Erythritol, powdered

1½ cups Almond Flour

½ cup Heavy Cream

2 tbsp Psyllium Husk Powder

1/3 cup Salted Butter

1/8 tsp Ground Clove

1 ½ tsp Baking Powder

½ tsp Orange Extract

1/8 tsp Ground Ginger

¼ tsp Liquid Stevia

¼ tsp Nutmeg

¼ tsp Allspice

For The Sugary Cinnamon Coating:

1/4 cup Erythritol

1/4 cup Butter, melted

1 tsp. Cinnamon

<u>Directions</u>

1. In a pan over medium-low heat, brown the butter, stirring occasionally.

2. In a spice grinder, powder the erythritol and clove twig (skip the twig if using pre-ground clove). Mix together all the dry ingredients.

3. Cool butter completely once browned. Add it to a bowl, add all the wet ingredients as well and mix with an electric mixer.

4. Sift half of the dry ingredients; add to the wet ingredients and mix. Repeat until the dough is formed.

5. Next, preheat the oven to 350F then divide out dough between 12 cupcake molds. Bake until edges are browned or for 20-25 minutes.

6. Melt 1/4 cup of butter in saucepan. Combine the cinnamon and desired sweetener.

7. Dip the cooled muffins into the butter, then into the "sugary" cinnamon mixture.

<u>Nutritional information per serving</u>

Calories 210, Fats 20.5g, Net Carb 2.5g, Protein 4g

Egg White Spinach Omelet

Servings: 1

<u>Ingredients</u>

1 Egg yolk

4-5 Egg whites

2 tbsp (30 ml) Almond milk, soymilk or coconut milk

½ or 1 Tomato

1 handful Shredded spinach

1 tbsp Purple onion

1 pinch Basil

Garlic (optional)

Olive oil cooking spray

<u>Directions:</u>

1. Chop the vegetables

2. Next, beat the eggs- egg whites& yolk. Add the almond milk and beat together.

3. Coat a small skillet with oil and sauté the vegetables quickly, just until soft.

4. Put the vegetables on the side, spray the pan again, put medium-low heat and pour the eggs.

5. Cook until the eggs are firm, add the vegetables on one side and fold the other half over top.

6. Add fruits to the plate and serve!

<u>Nutritional Information</u>

14

For the omelet only: Calories: 203, Fat: 5g, Protein: 20g, Carbs: 18g

Keto-Styled Scrambled Eggs

<u>Ingredients:</u>

1 tbsp of unsalted butter

3 Large Eggs

Coarse salt & freshly ground pepper

<u>Directions:</u>

1. Beat together the eggs using a fork.

2. In a medium nonstick pan, melt the butter over low heat.

3. Add the egg mixture.

4. Use a heatproof flexible spatula to pull the eggs gently to the center of the skillet. *Let the liquid parts run out under the perimeter*.

5. Cook, keep moving eggs around using the spatula for 2-3 minutes, just until the eggs are set.

6. Add salt and pepper to season. Serve hot.

<u>Nutritional Information:</u>

Calories 318, fat: 26.3 g, carbs: 1.8 g, protein: 17.4 g.

Bacon Frittata

Yields: 6 slices

Ingredients

4 large Bella Mushroom Caps

7 bacon slices

1 tbsp. olive oil

1/2 cup fresh basil, chopped

2 oz. Goat Cheese, Grated

4 oz. fresh mozzarella cheese, cubed

1 medium Red Bell Pepper

8-9 large Eggs

1/4 cup parmesan cheese, Grated

1/4 cup Heavy Cream

Salt& Pepper to taste

2 tbsp. Fresh Parsley (Garnish)

Directions:

1. Prep all the vegetables. Chop red pepper, basil, bacon and mushrooms roughly. Cube the mozzarella and then set aside.

2. Next, preheat oven to 350F.

3. Add olive oil in a hot pan. Once the first wisp of smoke becomes visible, add bacon immediately.

4. Leave the bacon to cook until browned. Add the red pepper and let it cook in the bacon fat until it is soft.

5. Meanwhile get a container, add eggs, heavy cream, parmesan cheese and black pepper to it. Mix eggs well with a whisk.

6. Once the red pepper softens, add the mushrooms to it, stirring well. The mushrooms should soak in the fat.

7. Add the fresh basil to the pan. Leave it to cook for a while then sprinkle the mozzarella cheese on top.

8. Next, pour eggs over them. Get the eggs under and around the ingredients in the pan by using a spoon to lift up the ingredients at the pan's bottom.

9. Add grated goat cheese over the top. Place in the oven for about 8 minutes. Broil the top in the broiler for 4-6 minutes more.

10. Use a spoon to remove from oven, pry the frittata edges away from the pan.

11. Once done, flip out of pan. Slice, serve and enjoy!

Nutritional Information Per Slice:

Calories 408, Fats, 31.2g, Net Carbs 2.4g & Protein19.2g

Hi-Fiber Coconut Coffee

Yield: 1 cup

<u>Ingredients</u>

2 tbsp (30g) Flaxseed, ground

2 tbsp (30g) Coconut flakes, unsweetened

1 tbsp Coconut oil

1/2 cup Black coffee, unsweetened

3-4 drops Liquid sweetener

<u>Directions:</u>

1. Mix the coconut flakes and flaxseed well. Add the coconut oil.

2. Pour the hot coffee over this mixture and mix. Depending on desired thickness, add more still water or coffee.

3. Add the sweetener to neutralize the bitterness of the coffee.

<u>Nutritional information</u>

Cal 277, fat 27, protein 4g, carbs 7g, fiber 5g, net carb 2g.

Easy Cheese& Onion Quiche

Yields: 2 quiches.

<u>Ingredients</u>

5-6 cups shredded Colby jack cheese and/or Muenster, divided

2 tbsp butter plus more

12 large eggs

2 cups heavy cream

1 large white onion, finely chopped

2 tsp dried thyme

1 tsp ground black pepper

1 tsp salt

<u>Directions:</u>

1. Preheat the oven to 350 degrees. Add the butter in a separate skillet and melt it over medium-low heat.

2. Now, add the vegetables, sautéing until onions are soft and translucent. Remove from heat and leave to cool.

3. Butter 2 quiche pans or deep pie pans of 10-inch. Put 2 cups of Muenster or shredded cheese in the bottom of the buttered pans.

4. In an even layer over the cheese, add half of the now-cooled vegetable mixture to each pan.

5. Pour cracked eggs into a large mixing bowl. Next, combine the cream and spices, whisking together until thoroughly mixed and frothy.

6. Pour ½ of the mixture over each pan of veggies and cheese. Gently distribute cheese and vegetables evenly into egg and cream using a fork.

7. Slide the quiche pans into the oven, leaving 1 inch of space between the pans. Bake for 20-25 minutes, until it is set and puffy and a little golden in the center.

8. Cut quiche into 6 equal-sized servings to make a total of 12 servings. Enjoy immediately or refrigerate or freeze. Refrigerate for up to 1 week and keep in the freezer for 2 weeks.

<u>Nutritional Information Per Serving</u>

Cal 382, fat 33, protein 16g, carbs 7g, fiber 1g, net carb 5g.

Keto Breakfast Blend

Yield: 1 jar

<u>Ingredients</u>

5 tbsp Coconut flakes, unsweetened (75g total)

7 tbsp Hemp seeds, (105g total)

5 tbsp Flaxseed, ground (80g)

2 tbsp Sesame, ground, (26g)

2 tbsp Cocoa, dark &unsweetened, (30g total)

2 tbsp Psyllium husk (18g total)

<u>Directions:</u>

1. Grind the sesame and flaxseed. (Grind the sesame seeds just enough to crack it, otherwise it will turn into a paste quickly).

2. Combine all the ingredients in a jar, shaking thoroughly. This should leave you with a jar containing 23 generous tablespoons of the mix, that is 1 tbsp = 1 serving.

3. Place in the refrigerator due to the high fat content of the sesame seeds and hemp.

4. Serve, softened with still water or black coffee. Add coconut oil to increase the fats intake. Also, it blends well with mascarpone cheese or cream.

Nutritional Information Per Serving

Cal49, fat 38, protein 2g, carbs 2.3g, fiber 1.7g, net carb 0.6. g.

Coco- Keto Cupcakes

Servings: 7

Ingredients

90g Coconut flakes, unsweetened

120g Vanilla-flavored protein powder

200ml Coconut milk, unsweetened,

4 tbsp Coconut oil,

2 tbsp Psyllium husk (12g)

 20g Dark chocolate min. 85% cocoa

Directions:

1. Mix the protein powder, the psyllium and the coconut flakes thoroughly in a medium sized bowl.

2. Add the coconut milk and the liquefied coconut oil into the mix and blend thoroughly.

3. Divide the batter into regular size cupcake forms of 7. Paper cupcake forms or silicone moulds can be used.

4. Crush the chocolate, melt it and decorate the cupcakes as desired.

5. Freeze the cupcakes for about 30 minutes to attain a more solid consistency.

6. Remove from the freezer. Store the cupcakes in the refrigerator.

<u>Nutritional Information Per Serving</u>

Cal 371, Fat 30.7g, Protein17.15g, Carbs10.1g, Fiber 5.85g, Net carbs4.25g

Super Egg Salad
Yield: 4 servings

Serving Size: 1/3 cup

A super simple, but tasty, low carb egg salad recipe.

<u>Ingredients</u>

2 tbsp mayonnaise

1 tsp lemon juice

1 tsp dijon mustard

1/4 tsp lite salt (for potassium)

6 eggs

Kosher salt & pepper to taste

<u>Directions:</u>

1. Gently place the eggs in a medium saucepan.

2. Pour cold water over the eggs, covering it by about 1 inch. Let it boil for 10 minutes. Remove and leave to cool.

3. Peel the eggs and add it to a food processor, pulsing until chopped.

4. Add the mustard, lemon juice, mayonnaise, salt and pepper then stir. Taste and adjust as needed.

5. Serve with lettuce leaves and if desired, bacon for wrapping.

Nutritional Information Per Serving:

Calories 166, fat14g, net carbs85g, protein10g

Chicharrones Con Huevos

Servings: 3

Ingredients

1 medium Avocado

1/4 cup Cilantro, chopped

5 large Eggs

4 slices Bacon

1 medium Tomato

2 medium Jalapeno Peppers, de-seeded

1.5 oz. Pork Rinds

1/4 medium Onion

Salt and Pepper to Taste

Directions:

1. Cook the bacon and transfer to paper towel. Keep the bacon fat in the pan.

2. Next, cook the pork rinds in the bacon fat and add the diced vegetables.

3. Add cilantro once the onions are almost translucent and then mix together.

4. Now add pre-scrambled eggs, leave to cook and stir once.

5. Cube avocado and fold into eggs. Enjoy!

<u>Nutritional Information Per Serving:</u>

Calories 508, Fats 43g, Net Carbs 5g & Protein 24.7g

Butter Hardboiled Eggs

Servings: 1

<u>Ingredients</u>

2 whole Eggs

30g Butter

1 tbsp Mascarpone

Salt &pepper to taste

<u>Directions:</u>

1. Hard boil the eggs in a pot. Add a pinch of salt to it so the eggs will peel better once done.

2. Wash the boiled eggs with cold water. Peel and chop into a large cup.

3. Next, add the mascarpone cheese and butter while the eggs are still hot, mixing well. Season with salt and pepper.

<u>Nutritional Information Per Serving:</u>

Calories 430, fat41g, net carbs1g, protein14g

Chia Sunrise Custard

2 tbsp chia seeds

1/4 cup heavy cream

1 egg yolk

20 drops liquid stevia extract (10 drops each French Vanilla & English Toffee)

1/2 cup water

1 pinch salt

Directions:

1. Put the chia seeds in a small bowl, add the water and stir. Keep refrigerated overnight.

2. Remove from fridge in the morning. Use a fork to stir and break up clumps.

3. Pour the cream into a measuring cup. Add the egg yolk alone and stir together with a fork.

4. Stir in the salt and liquid stevia extract.

5. Pour the mixture into the chia seeds, stirring thoroughly again to break up any clumps. (Use a glass custard cup so it's easy to see through any stubborn clumps of chia seed).

6. Put the chia custard in the microwave, set on power 5 and leave for 1 minute. Stir, leave for another 1 minute and then turn it off.

7. Enjoy with sprinkled sugar-free chocolate chips, pancake syrup or a cinnamon.

Nutritional Information Per Serving

Calories 408; Fat 36g, Protein9g; Carb14g; Fiber10g

Blackberry Breakfast Pudding
Servings: 2

Ingredients

1/4 tsp. Baking Powder

1/4 cup Coconut Flour

2 tbsp. Coconut Oil

5 large Egg Yolks

2 tbsp. Butter

2 tsp. Lemon Juice

2 tbsp. Heavy Cream

10 drops Liquid Stevia

Zest 1 Lemon

2 tbsp. Erythritol

1/4 cup Blackberries

Direction

1. Preheat the oven to 350F.

2. Beat the egg yolks until it is pale in color. Add stevia and erythritol, beating again until fully mixed.

3. Add heavy cream, lemon zest, butter, lemon juice and coconut oil. Beat until well combined.

4. Sift the dry ingredients and add to the wet ingredients, mixing well again.

5. Distribute the batter between two ramekins. Crush 2 tbsp. Blackberries slightly with your fingers and push into each ramekin.

6. Bake for about 25 minutes. Allow to cool and enjoy!

Nutritional Information Per Serving

Calories 477; Fat 43.5g, Protein9g; Carb5.5g

Kitchen Frittata

Servings: 8 slices

Ingredients

3 chicken Sausages, chopped

3 cups Raw Spinach, chopped

2 ½ cup Mushrooms, chopped

1 ½ cup cheddar cheese

2 tsp. hot sauce

10 Large Eggs

1/2 tsp. Mrs. Dash Table Blend

1 tbsp. Ranch Dressing

Directions

1. Preheat oven to 400F.

2. Cook sausages on medium high heat in a cast iron skillet to get crisp and nice.

3. Add the spinach and mushrooms to the skillet and leave to cook down.

4. Crack the eggs into a bowl. Add the hot sauce, ranch and spices. Combine well.

5. Once the spinach is cooked down, add the eggs and cheese and thoroughly mix it in.

6. Put the skillet in the oven for 10 minutes. Broil for 3-4 minutes more.

<u>Nutritional Information Per Serving</u>

Calories240, Fats17.8g, Net Carbs 2.2g, Protein19.9g.

Cinnamon Roll Cereal

Servings: 6

<u>Ingredients</u>

1 cup crushed pecans

1/3 cup chia seed

1/3 cup flax seed

½ cup cauliflower, riced

3 ½ cups coconut milk

3 oz. cream cheese

3 tbsp. Butter

1 ½ tsp. cinnamon

1/2 tsp. vanilla

1/4 cup heavy cream

1 tsp. maple flavor

1/4 tsp. nutmeg

1/4 tsp. allspice

10-15 drops Liquid Stevia

3 tbsp. Erythritol, powdered

1/8 tsp. Xanthan Gum (optional)

Directions

1. In a food processor, rice cauliflower and then set aside. Start to heat coconut milk in a skillet over medium heat.

2. Crush the pecans; add it to skillet to toast over low heat.

3. Add the cauliflower to the coconut milk and bring to a boil. Reduce to simmer, add the spices and combine.

4. Grind the erythritol and add it to the skillet. Add the chia seed, stevia and flax. Mix thoroughly together.

5. Add butter, cream cheese and cream to the skillet and mix again. If desired, add xanthan gum to make it a bit thicker.

Nutritional Information Per Serving

Calories398, Fats37.7g, Net Carbs 3.1g, Protein8.8g.

Coconut Custard Macadamia Nut

It's a perfect keto treat - well almost!

<u>Ingredients</u>

4 Large Eggs

1 cup unsweetened coconut milk

1/3 cup heavy cream

1/3 Cup Erythritol

1/3 cup macadamia nut butter

1 tsp. Vanilla Extract

1 tsp. Liquid Stevia

<u>Directions</u>

1. Preheat oven to 325F. Combine all ingredients in a mixing bowl and whisk gently so as not to over-aerate the eggs.

2. Fill a small pan with an inch of water. Place 4 ramekins in it and fill them with the custard mixture in equal proportions.

3. Bake until a knife comes out clean or for 40 minutes.

4. Let it cool for 30 to 45 minutes. Serve and enjoy!

4. Wrap leftover with plastic and refrigerate.

<u>Nutritional Information Per Serving</u>

Calories275, Fats26.2g, Net Carbs 2.5g, Protein6.2g.

Crunchy Bacon Baskets

Servings: 4

<u>Ingredients</u>

4 cups spinach

12 bacon slices

2 tbsp. heavy cream

4 large eggs

2/3 cup cheddar cheese

1 tsp. pepper

1 tbsp. olive oil

<u>Directions</u>

1. Preheat the oven to 350F.

2. Next, make bacon weave. Cut the weaves into quarters.

3. Toss a cupcake tray, use a foil to cover in the 4 corners and then carefully lay bacon weave on the foil.

4. Bake for about 50 minutes. Bring it out; let it cool for 10 minutes then switch the oven to broil.

5. Get a bowl, break 2 eggs into it then add heavy cream and beat.

6. In a pan, heat the olive oil and cook down the spinach. Add black pepper.

7. Once spinach is cooked, add the eggs, turn heat to low and cook.

8. Fill the bacon baskets with the spinach and egg mixture. Top with cheese.

9. Place in oven; broil until cheese forms a nice crust. Take it out and serve.

Nutritional Information Per Serving

Calories325, Fats26g, Net Carbs 1.5g, Protein19.8g.

Seafood Breakfast Spread
Yields: 12 ounces of spread

Ingredients

2 ounces of full fat mayonnaise

4.5 oz. cream cheese

½ tsp black pepper

1 tsp lemon juice

½ tsp dried dill

4.25 ounces canned pink salmon, boneless & skinless

3 ounces shrimp, boiled or steamed

1 tsp sea salt

Directions

1. Put the cream cheese in a glass bowl and place in the microwave to soften for 50-60 seconds.

2. Remove. Add mayonnaise and whisk until smooth. Add spices and lemon juice then whisk again.

3. Add the shrimp and salmon to a food processor bowl fitted with an S-blade.

4. Next, add the cream cheese mixture and then process to a spread consistency for about 30 - 60 seconds.

5. Eat immediately or refrigerate until ready to serve.

Serve wrapped in romaine lettuce leaves or with almond flour mini tart shells.

Nutritional Information Per Serving

Calories95, Fats8g, Net Carbs 6g, Protein5g.

KETO LUNCH RECIPES

Cauliflower Casserole
Servings: 10

Ingredients

12 Chicken Thighs (4 Oz. Each)

1 Head Cauliflower, chopped (30 Oz.)

8 Oz Monterey Jack Cheese, Shredded

8 Oz Cheddar Cheese, Shredded

6 Green Onions (75g total)

1 Medium Onion (162g)

6 Thick Bacon Slices, Cut

1 Medium Green Pepper (147g)

1 Tablespoon Minced Garlic

8 Oz Cream Cheese

4 Oz Heavy Cream

Salt and Pepper to taste

Directions

1. Get a casserole dish; add chicken thighs to it, add salt and pepper and some water to about mid thigh. Cook for 60 minutes at 350 degrees.

2. Cook bacon in the oven at 450 degrees for 15 to 20minutes

3. Cooked chopped cauliflower in the microwave, placing on vegetable setting.

4. Chop up peppers and onions and pan fry.

5. If baking the chicken in the oven, chop up the cooked chicken into a bowl.

6. Add all the ingredients, keeping aside 2 Oz Monterey Jack and 2 Oz Cheddar.

7. Add mixture into a greased casserole dish. Top with the remaining cheese.

8. Finally, cover with foil, cook at 350 degrees for 25 minutes. Remove foil and cook for another 5 minutes.

Nutrition Information Per Serving

Calories: 516, Fat: 34, Carbs: 9, Fiber: 3, Protein: 44

Tomato Pesto Cake
Yields: 1

Ingredients

For the base:

1 Large Egg

2 Tbsp. Almond Flour

2 Tbsp. Butter

1/2 tsp. Baking Powder

For the flavor:

1 Tbsp. Almond Flour

5 tsp. Sun Dried Tomato Pesto

Pinch Salt

1. Mix together all ingredients.

2. Microwave on high for 75 seconds (power level 10).

3. To take the mug cake out, slam cup lightly against plate.

4. Add extra tomato pesto. Serve!

Nutritional Information Per Serving

Calories 365, Fat 28g, Total Carb 20g, Fiber 1g, Protein 9g

Avocado Chicken Casserole
Servings: 6

Ingredients

4 Small Avocados, peeled

8 Boneless Chicken Thighs, cooked

1 Medium Pepper

1 Medium Onion

8 Oz. Cheddar Cheese

8 Oz. Sour Cream

1 Tbsp Frank's Red Hot

Salt & Pepper to taste

Directions

1. Preheat oven to 350 F. Bake the cooked chicken thighs for 1 and half hours, cover with some water and pan fry until the juices are clear.

2. Cut the peeled avocado in half and then slice into thin strips.

3. Line the bottom of a greased baking dish with avocado slices. Keep any extra.

4. Cut the onions and peppers into strips and pan-fry until caramelized.

5. Get a large bowl. Place the chicken in it and flake apart.

6. Add the rest of the ingredients, as well as any extra avocado and then mix.

7. Spoon the mixture over the slices of avocado. Bake for 20 minutes. Remove and serve.

Nutrition Information Per Serving

Calories: 549, Fat: 40g, Carbs: 13g, Protein: 39g, Fiber: 7g

Marinated Pork Chops

Servings: 10

Ingredients

18 Pork Chops (approx. 4.46lbs)

½ Cup Apple Cider Vinegar

4 tbsp Soy Sauce

½ tsp Ginger

½ tsp Pepper

½ Cup Splenda

Directions

1. Add all the ingredients to a food processor (except the pork chops) and mix

2. Grease a pan. Place the pork chops in it then pour the marinade over it.

3. Cook at 350 degrees for up to 60 minutes. Flip after 30 minutes.

5. Chop up pork chops into pieces and divide into 10 lunch servings.

Nutritional Information Per Serving

Calories: 323 Fat: 14 Carb: 1 Fiber: 0 Protein: 46

Crispy-Fried Wings

Servings: 2

Serving size: 6 wings

Ingredients

12 chicken wings, raw &thawed

4 tbsp unsalted butter

4 tbsp Frank's Red Hot

Directions

1. Preheat the fryer oil to 275. Dry the wings and fry for 15 minutes

2. Let wings cool to room temperature.

3. Preheat the fryer to 375 and pat wings dry.

4. Fry for another 6 minutes or until skin is taut and golden brown.

5. If desired, mix melted butter and Frank's Red Hot together.

6. Toss the crispy fried wings in the sauce. Serve!

<u>Nutritional Information Per Serving</u>

Calories: 686, Fat: 55, Carb 0, Fiber: 0, Protein: 42

Peanut Shrimp Curry

Servings: 2.

<u>Ingredients</u>

6 oz. Pre-cooked Shrimp

2 tbsp Green Curry Paste

1 cup Coconut Milk

1 cup Vegetable Stock

3 tbsp Cilantro, chopped

5 oz. Broccoli Florets

1 tbsp. Peanut Butter

2 tbsp. Coconut Oil

Juice of 1/2 Lime

1 tbsp. Soy Sauce coconut aminos

1 medium Spring Onion, chopped

1 tsp. roasted garlic, crushed

1/2 tsp. Turmeric

1 tsp. Fish Sauce

1 tsp. Minced Ginger

1/4 tsp. Xanthan Gum

1/2 cup Sour Cream (for topping)

Directions

1. Add the coconut oil to a pan and set on medium heat.

2. Once hot, add garlic, ginger and spring onion. Let it cook then add fish sauce, peanut butter, turmeric, soy sauce and 1 tbsp of green curry paste.

3. Stir together then add coconut milk and vegetable broth.

4. Add xanthan gum and mix well then add broccoli and mix thoroughly.

5. Add cilantro and shrimp to the pan and combine well.

6. Let it cook for about 5 minutes.

7. Serve with a spoonful of sour cream over the top!

Nutritional Information Per Serving

Calories 455, Fats: 31.5g, Net Carbs: 8.9g, Protein: 27g.

Grilled Cheese Sandwich

Yield: 1

<u>Ingredients</u>

For the bun:

2 tbsp almond flour

2 large eggs

2 tbsp soft butter

1 ½ tbsp Psyllium Husk Powder

½ tsp Baking Powder

Fillings & Extras:

2 Oz. cheddar cheese

1 tbsp butter, for frying

<u>Directions</u>

1. Mix together the bun ingredients in a container and continue to mix until it thickens.

2. Pour the mixture into container and level off. If necessary, clean the sides.

3. Microwave for 90 seconds. If undone by this time, keep increasing it by 15 seconds.

4. Once cooked, remove and slice in half.

5. Put the cheese between the bun. In a pan, heat butter over medium heat then fry the grilled cheese to desired texture.

<u>Nutritional Information Per Sandwich</u>

Calories 793, Fats 70g, Net Carbs 4.7g & Protein 29g

Yummy Chicken Satay

Yields: 3

<u>Ingredients</u>

4 tbsp soy sauce

1 tsp. Minced Garlic

1 lb. Ground Chicken

3 tbsp peanut butter

2 tsp. Chili Paste

1/3 Yellow Pepper, sliced

2 Spring Onions, chopped

1 tbsp. Erythritol

2 tsp. Sesame Oil

1 tbsp. Rice Vinegar

1/4 tsp. Paprika

1/4 tsp. Cayenne

Juice of 1/2 Lime

<u>Directions</u>

1. Heat the sesame oil in a pan on medium-high heat.

2. Brown the ground chicken. Add all other ingredients to it. Mix well and keep cooking.

3. Once cooked, add spring onions and yellow pepper.

4. Enjoy!

<u>Nutritional Information Per Serving</u>

Calories 393, Fats: 23g, Net Carbs: 3.7g, Protein: 35g.

Beanless Chili Con Carne

Servings: 5

<u>Ingredients</u>

1 lb Hot Italian Sausage

1 lb Ground Beef

1 Large Green Pepper

1 Medium White Onion

2 tbsp Curry Powder

1 Large Yellow Pepper

1 Can Tomato Sauce

2 tbsp. Cumin

2 tbsp Chili Powder

1 tbsp Butter

1 tbsp Organic Coconut Oil

1 tbsp Minced Garlic

1 tsp Onion Powder

1 tsp. Freshly Ground Black Pepper

1 tsp. Salt

Directions

1. Dice peppers and the onion evenly. Mince garlic finely.

2. Set a big pan to medium-high heat. Add the coconut oil and butter and melt.

4. Add the peppers, onion and minced garlic to pan. Let them sauté down and stir often.

5. Set a pot on medium heat, add the ground beef and hot sausage, cook until browned, add salt and pepper to taste.

6. Add the peppers, onion and garlic to the pot along with the sausage and ground beef. Mix together.

7. Add tomato sauce, chili powder and onion powder and cook for 20 minutes.

8. Add cumin and curry powder, cook for 10 more minutes, stirring often.

9. Depending on desired thickness, let it simmer for 45 minutes to 2 hours.

Nutritional Information Per Serving

Calories 415, Fats: 25g, Net Carbs: 6g

Spicy Keto Chili

Servings: 8

Ingredients

8 Cups Spinach

2 lbs. Ground Beef

2 Green Bell Peppers

1 Cup Tomato Sauce

2/3 Medium Onion

1 tbsp. Cumin

1 tbsp. Olive Oil

1 Tbsp. Chili Powder

1 tbsp. Curry Powder

1 tsp. Garlic Powder

2 tsp. Cayenne Pepper

1 tsp. Xanthan Gum

Directions

1. Slice bell peppers and onions. Brown the ground beef in a pot.

2. Meanwhile, sauté vegetables in olive oil in a separate pan.

3. Add spices to the ground beef and mix well. Season the vegetables and set to medium heat.

4. Add spinach to ground beef. Cook down and stir in then add tomato sauce, mixing well and cooking for 10 minutes.

5. Turn vegetables off. Add onions and peppers to the beef mixture and stir.

6. Add xanthan gum and stir until thickened. Cook for 15 minutes.

7. Serve hot with sour cream or cheese on top.

Nutritional Information Per Serving

Calories 357, Fats: 22g, Net Carbs: 4.5g, Protein: 31g.

Basil Fresh Bell Pepper Pizza
Yields: 2 pizzas

Ingredients

For the Pizza Base:

½ cup Almond Flour

6 oz. Mozzarella Cheese

2 tbsp. Cream Cheese

2 tbsp. Psyllium Husk

1 large Egg

2 tbsp. Fresh Parmesan Cheese

1 tsp. Italian Seasoning

½ tsp. Pepper

½ tsp. Salt

For the Toppings:

4 oz. Cheddar Cheese, Shredded

2/3 medium Bell Pepper

1/4 cup Rao's Tomato Sauce

1 medium Vine Tomato

2-3 tbsp. Fresh Chopped Basil

Directions

1. Preheat the oven to 400F.

2. Next, microwave mozzarella cheese until fully melted and pliable or for 40-50 seconds

3. Add the remaining pizza ingredients to the cheese (except the toppings) and mix together with your hands.

4. Use a rolling pin or your hands to flatten the dough then form a circle.

5. Bake for about 10 minutes then remove pizza from oven.

6. Top pizza with the toppings, baking for 8-10 minutes more.

6. Remove from the oven. Let it cool and serve.

Nutritional Information Per Serving

Calories 410, Fats: 31.3g, Net Carbs: 5.3g, Protein: 24.8g.

Hot Jalapeno Poppers
Yield: 8

<u>Ingredients</u>

8 slices Bacon

8 medium Jalapeno Peppers

1/4 cup Mozzarella Cheese

5 oz. Cream Cheese

1/2 tsp. Mrs. Dash Table Blend

1/4 tsp. Salt

1/4 tsp. Pepper

<u>Directions</u>

1. Preheat oven to 400F. Next, slice jalapenos in half; scrape out the insides of the peppers.

2. Mix together mozzarella cheese, cream cheese and desired spices in a bowl.

3. Pack the cream cheese mixture into peppers. Place the other half of pepper on top, close peppers up again.

4. Next, wrap each pepper in 1 bacon slice, beginning from the bottom then working up.

5. Bake for 20 to 25 minutes, broil for another 2 to 3 minutes. Serve.

<u>Nutritional Information Per Serving</u>

Calories 182, Fats: 16.5g, Net Carbs: 1.3 g, Protein: 4.8g.

Crunchy Skin Pork Shoulder

Servings: 20

Size: 6 oz.

Ingredients

8 lbs. Pork Shoulder

1 tsp. Onion Powder

1 tsp. Garlic Powder

2 tsp. Oregano

1 tsp. Black Pepper

3 1/2 tbsp. Salt

Directions

1. Wash the pork, dry it and let it come to room temperature.

2. Preheat oven to 250 F. Rub spices and salt over the pork shoulder.

3. Place onto a wire rack over a foil-covered baking sheet. Bake for 8-10 hours, depending on size or until the internal temperature is about 190F.

4. Take out meat from oven, cover with foil and let it rest for 15 minutes.

5. Meanwhile, heat oven to 500F. Take out foil and roast the pork for another 20 minutes, 500F in total and rotating every 5 minutes.

6. Let the pork rest for about 20 minutes. Cut and serve.

Nutritional Information Per Serving

Calories 461, Fats: 36.7g, Net Carbs: 0.2 g, Protein: 30.3g.

Chicken Curry With Paneer Butter

Servings: 4

<u>Ingredients</u>

7 Oz Paneer Packet, cut into pieces

3lbs Chicken Thighs (with bone in)

1 Cup Crushed Tomatoes

4 Tbsp. Butter

1/2 Cup Heavy Whipping Cream

1 Tbsp. Olive Oil

1 1/2 tsp. Garlic Paste

2 tsp. Coconut Oil

1 tsp. Coriander Powder

1 1/2 tsp. Ginger Paste

1/2 tsp. Paprika

1 tsp. Garam Masala

5 Sprigs Cilantro

1/2 tsp. Red Chili Powder

1/2 tsp. Kashmiri Mirch

1 Cup Water

1 tsp. Freshly Ground Black Pepper

1 tsp. Salt

<u>Directions</u>

1. Preheat the oven to 375 F. Rub entire chicken thighs with olive oil, salt & pepper to taste.

2. Put on a cookie sheet and roast for 20- 25 minutes. Add the coconut oil and butter to a pan on medium heat. Let the butter brown.

3. Once butter has browned, add garlic paste ginger then sauté for 2 minutes.

4. Add the crushed tomato, coriander powder, paprika, red chili powder and salt, mixing well and allowing to simmer until oil becomes visible at the top.

5. Mix paneer gently into the sauce. Pour in water and simmer for 5 minutes.

6. Next, turn heat to medium low, add cream and stir to mix, simmering until it comes to a boil again.

7. Take out chicken and separate it from the bone (it shouldn't be completely cooked).

8. Now add the chicken to sauce and mix thoroughly. Simmer for another 5-10 minutes.

9. Garnish with cilantro. Serve hot

<u>Nutritional Information Per Serving</u>

Calories: 489, Fats: 44g, Net Carbs: 4g.

Crispy Keto Nuggets

Servings: 2

Serving size: 5 nuggets

Ingredients

1 (4 Oz.) Chicken Breast, cooked

½ Oz. Parmesan, Grated

½ tsp Baking Powder

2 Tbsp Almond Flour

1 egg

1 Tbsp Water

Directions

1. Heat deep fryer to 375 degrees. Cut cooked chicken breast into cubes.

2. Mix the almond flour, parmesan and baking powder.

3. Next, add the egg, whisk and add the water and whisk.

4. Coat the chicken breasts by rolling them in the batter then drop them into the frying oil with a fork.

5. (Ensure they do not stick to the bottom, flip them with a fork every minute or so if necessary).

6. Cook 5 minutes or until the batter turns golden brown.

Nutritional Information Per Serving

Calories: 166, Fat: 8g, Carb: 2g, Fiber: 1, Protein: 23

Oriental Keto Pork Chops

Servings: 2

<u>Ingredients</u>

4 boneless pork chops

1 stalk lemongrass (peeled &diced)

1 medium star anise

1 tbsp fish sauce

4 garlic cloves, halved

1 tbsp almond flour

½ tbsp. Sambal chili paste

½ tbsp. sugar free ketchup

1 ½ tsp soy sauce

½ tsp five-spice

1 tsp sesame oil

½ tsp peppercorns

<u>Directions</u>

1. Place pork chops on a flat surface then pound to ½ inch thick.

2. In a blender or mortar, grind the star anise and peppercorns to a fine powder.

3. Add the garlic and lemongrass and blend or pound until a puree forms. Add soy sauce, fish sauce, five spice powder, sesame oil and mix well.

4. Get a tray, put the pork chops in it, add marinade and turn to coat. Cover it and marinate at room temperature for 1 to 2 hours.

5. Heat a pan to high. Coat the pork chops lightly with almond flour and add to the pan, searing them about 2 minutes per side and turning once.

6. Place onto a cutting board then cut each pork chop into many strips.

7. For the sauce, mix the sugar-free ketchup and Sambal chili paste together.

8. Enjoy your delicious meal!

<u>Nutritional Information Per Serving</u>

Calories: 272, Fat: 9.5g, Carb: 6g, Protein: 34g

Enchilada Chicken Soup
Servings: 4

<u>Ingredients</u>

3 Tbsp Olive Oil

1 medium Red Bell Pepper, diced

3 stalks Celery, diced

4 cups Chicken Broth

2 tsp. Garlic, minced

1 cup Diced Tomatoes

6 oz. Chicken, shredded

8 oz. Cream Cheese

2 tsp. Cumin

1 tsp. Chili Powder

1 tsp Oregano

1/2 cup Cilantro, chopped

1/2 tsp. Cayenne Pepper

1/2 medium Lime, juiced

Directions

1. In a pan, heat oil and add pepper and celery. Once the celery is soft, add the tomatoes and cook for 2 to 3 minutes.

2. Add spices to pan then mix together thoroughly.

3. Pour in the cilantro and chicken broth, bring to a boil, reduce to low and simmer for 20 minutes.

4. Now add cream cheese and then bring to a boil once more. Once it boils, set heat to low and then simmer for 25 minutes.

5. Add shredded chicken to a pot and then pour juice lime over the top. Mix everything together.

6. Enjoy with an extra sprinkling of cilantro sour cream or shredded cheese!

Nutritional Information Per Serving

Calories 345, Fats 31.3g, Net Carbs 6g & Protein13.3g

Spinach Salad With Spicy Bacon Dressing

Yields: 2

Ingredients

4 slices bacon

1 bag fresh baby spinach

2 hard boiled eggs, chopped

1/4 cup chopped onion

1 pkg Splenda

1/4 cup vinegar

Salt & pepper

Directions

1. Cook bacon, let it drain on paper towel. Keep bacon grease in pan.

2. Add pepper, splenda and vinegar to bacon grease, stirring and heating slowly until boiling.

3. Tear the spinach into salad sized pieces, toss with crumbled bacon, egg and onion.

4. Pour on hot dressing immediately and toss lightly.

Net carbs: 5 grams per serving

KETO DINNER RECIPES

Bacon Cheeseburger Soup

Servings: 5

Ingredients

5 Bacon slices

12 oz. Ground Beef

3 oz. Cream Cheese

3 cups Beef Broth

2 tbsp. Butter

1/2 tsp. Garlic Powder

2 tsp. Brown Mustard

1/2 tsp. Onion Powder

1 ½ tsp. Kosher Salt

½ tsp. Black Pepper

1 tsp. Cumin

1/2 tsp. Red Pepper Flakes

1 tsp. Chili Powder

1 medium Dill Pickle, diced

2 1/2 tbsp. Tomato Paste

1 cup Cheddar Cheese, Shredded

1/2 cup Heavy Cream

Directions

1. In a pan, cook bacon until it is crispy then set it aside.

2. Add the ground beef in the bacon fat. Cook until browned on both sides.

3. Put the beef in a pot, moving it to the sides. Next, add spices and butter to the pan and leave for 30-45 seconds.

4. Add tomato paste, beef broth, pickles and cheese to the pot. Let it cook until melted.

5. Cover the pot, turn heat to low and cook for 20 to 30 minutes.

6. Turn off stove; finish with crumbled bacon and heavy cream. Stir and serve.

Nutritional Information Per Serving

Calories 572, Fats 48.6g, Net Carbs 3.4g & Protein 23.4g

Cauliflower Soup With Bacon& Cheddar

Servings: 6

Ingredients

4 Slices Bacon

1 Cauliflower Head, diced (1.016 kg)

1 Medium Onion, diced (169 g)

12 Oz. Aged Cheddar (3+ years), shredded

2 Tbsp Olive Oil

1 Oz Parmesan Cheese

1 tsp Ground Thyme

¼ Cup Heavy Cream

3 Cups Chicken Broth

1 Tbsp Minced Garlic

<u>Directions</u>

1. Place diced cauliflower on a foil-lined sheet then drizzle with olive oil.

2. Season the cauliflower and bacon with salt and pepper and cook for 35 minutes at 375 degrees or until bacon is crisp.

3. Fry diced onion in the bacon grease then add the garlic and thyme, cooking for 30 seconds to 1 minute.

4. Add the cauliflower and chicken broth, cover and simmer for 20 minutes.

5. Use an immersion blender to blend cauliflower into a soup.

6. Now add the cheese and blend again.

7. Add the cream and bacon and combine thoroughly with a spoon

<u>Nutritional Information Per Serving</u>

Calories: 337, Fat: 25, Carb: 11, Fiber: 4, Protein: 18

Pork Kabobs In Sunflower Butter

Servings: 4

<u>Ingredients</u>

2 tsp Hot Sauce

3 tbsp Sunflower Butter

1 tbsp Soy Sauce

½ tsp Crushed Red Pepper

1 tbsp Minced Garlic

1 Lb Pork Kabob Squares

1 medium Green Pepper, chopped

<u>Directions</u>

1. Place the marinade ingredients into a food processor then mix until smooth.

2. Place the cut pork in a non-metal bowl. Next, mix together the pork and marinade and let it marinate for 1 hour or up to 24 hours.

3. Thread the pork and chopped green pepper onto metal skewers.

4. Broil for 5 minutes on high on each side or until internal temperature reaches 145 degrees

<u>Nutritional Information Per Serving</u>

Calories: 200, Fat: 8g, Carb: 5g, Protein: 24g

Stuffed Roasted Chicken With Gravy

Servings: 8

<u>Ingredients</u>

10 strips bacon

1 Whole Chicken, gutted (3 lbs.)

4 sprigs Fresh Thyme

1 small Lime

1 tbsp. Grain Mustard

1 medium Lemon

Salt & Pepper to Taste

<u>Directions</u>

1. Preheat oven to 500F.

2. Next, season chicken with salt and pepper. Stuff it with thyme, lime and lemon.

3. Wrap the bacon over bird skin and season the bacon with salt & pepper.

4. Next, place bird in roasting pan; put it inside the oven for about 15 minutes. Reduce temperature to 350F then bake for 40-50 minutes more.

5. Remove the chicken and place in foil. Put the pan juices in a pan and then bring to a boil.

6. Add mustard to the pan liquids, mix well and reduce slightly

7. using an immersion blender, blend the sauce in the pan.

8. Serve the chicken with gravy.

<u>Nutritional Information Per Serving</u>

Calories: 376, Fat:29.8g, Carb: 1.5g, Protein: 24.5g

Delicious Pork Tacos
Servings: 3

<u>Ingredients</u>

1 lb. Pork Shoulder, cooked

1 cup Romaine Lettuce, shredded

1 tbsp. Olive Oil

1/4 tsp. Onion Powder

1/2 tsp. Chipotle Powder

1/4 tsp. Pepper

1/4 tsp. Oregano

1/4 tsp. Garlic Powder

1 medium Jalapeno Pepper

3/4 medium Yellow Pepper

6 thin Flax Tortillas

1 tbsp. Olive Oil

1/2 tsp. Salt

<u>Directions</u>

1. Make flax tortillas.

2. Chop pork up into cubes

3. In a tightly rolled plastic bag, marinade pork in oil and spices for 30 to 45 minutes.

4. Chop vegetables, sauté in olive oil on high heat until cooked then set aside.

5. Cook pork on high until well browned.

6. Assemble tacos with vegetables, pork and lettuce. Top with sour cream and enjoy!

Per 2 Tacos With Fillings:

Calories718, Fats67.6g, Net Carbs3.2g, and Protein 35.7g

Rich Pork Chops
Servings: 4

Ingredients

Pork Chops, Cut (3.67 lbs, 2" thick)

3 Oz. Bleu Cheese

3 Bacon Slices

60 g Green Onion

3 Oz. Feta Cheese

2 Oz. Cream Cheese

Salt, pepper & garlic powder to taste

<u>Directions</u>

1. Place bacon in a skillet and cook, reserving the grease then setting the bacon aside.

2. In a bowl, mix together the feta and bleu cheeses. Add the green onions and bacon and mix.

3. Next, add the cream cheese. Mix until combined.

4. Gently slice open the non- fat side of the pork chops and stuff it with cheese mixture. Close opening with a toothpick.

6. Season exterior of pork chops with salt, pepper and garlic powder.

7. Sear over high heat, with bacon grease in pan for 1.5 minutes per side.

8. Place chops to a greased pan then cook for 55 minutes at 350 degrees.

9. Take out pork chops. Let it rest for 3 minutes then serve.

<u>Nutritional Information Per Serving</u>

Calories: 778, Fat: 38, Carb: 2, Fiber: 1, Protein: 102

Zesty Chicken Nuggets With Avocado Sauce

Servings: 4

<u>Ingredients</u>

For the Nuggets:

1 large Egg

24oz Chicken Thighs, cut

1/4 tsp. Chili Powder

1/4 cup Almond Meal

1.5 oz Pork Rinds

Zest 1 Lime

1/4 cup Flax Meal

1/4 tsp. Paprika

1/4 tsp. Salt

1/4 tsp. Pepper

1/8 tsp. Onion Powder

1/8 tsp. Cayenne Pepper

1/8 tsp. Garlic Powder

 For The Sauce:

1/2 medium Hass Avocado

1/2 cup Mayonnaise

1 tbsp. Lime Juice

1/2 tsp. Red Chili Flakes

1/8 tsp. Cumin

1/4 tsp. Garlic Powder

1. Dry the chicken and slice into bite-size pieces.

2. Pulse all the crust ingredients in a food processor.

3. Put the crumbs and a whisked egg in 2 separate bowls.

4. Dip the chicken in the whisked egg, then dip in the crust and lay it on a greased baking sheet.

5. Next, bake for 15-18 minutes at 400F. Make the sauce by mixing all ingredients together.

Nutritional Information Per Serving

Calories: 613, Fat: 50g, Carb: 1.8, Protein: 38.8

Hot Sausage & Pepper Soup
Servings: 4

Ingredients

1 Can Tomatoes with Jalapenos

1.4 lb. Hot Italian Sausage, cut into chunks

2 Cups Beef Stock

6 Cups Raw Spinach

1 Red Bell Pepper

1 Green Bell Pepper

1/2 Medium Onion

2 tsp. Chili powder

2 tsp. Minced Garlic

2 tsp. Cumin

1 tsp. Italian Seasoning

1/2 tsp. Kosher Salt

Directions

1. Cook sausage all the way through.

2. Add sliced tomatoes, peppers, spices and beef stock to slow cooker. Put the sausage on top then mix well.

3. Fry the garlic and onions, add to slow cooker when translucent.

4. Next, add spinach on top and let it cook on high for 3 hours.

5. after 3 hours, stir and cook on low for 2 hours more.

Nutritional Information Per Serving

Calories 385, Fats 27g, Net Carbs 6.9g &Protein24g

Zesty Pepperoni Pizza

Yields: 6 slices.

<u>Ingredients</u>

For the Pizza Base:

2 cups Mozzarella Cheese

1 tbsp. Psyllium Husk Powder

3/4 cup Almond Flour

3 tbsp. Cream Cheese

1 tbsp. Italian Seasoning

1 large Egg

1/2 tsp. Salt

1/2 tsp. Pepper

 For the Toppings:

16 slices Pepperoni

1/2 cup Rao's Tomato Sauce

1 cup Mozzarella Cheese

Sprinkled Oregano (optional)

<u>Directions</u>

1. Microwave the mozzarella cheese until fully melted, then add all base ingredients (except the olive oil) and combine well.

2. Knead the dough into a ball, spread out into a circle with the olive oil on the outside of the dough.

3. Next, bake crust under 400F for 10 minutes. Take it out from the oven, flip and bake for another 2-4 minutes.

4. Top the crust with desired toppings and bake for 3-5 minutes more.

5. Let it cool for a while, slice, serve and enjoy.

<u>Nutritional Information Per Serving</u>

Calories 335, Fats 27g, Net Carbs 3.2g &Protein18.2g

Asian Crockpot Pork Hock

Yields: 2

<u>Ingredients</u>

1 lb Pork Hock

1/3 Cup Soy Sauce

1/4 Cup Rice Vinegar

1 Tbsp. Butter or Coconut Oil

1/4 Cup Splenda

2 Cloves Garlic, Crushed

1/3 Cup Shaoxing Cooking Wine

1/3 Medium Onion

Handful of Shitake Mushrooms

1 tsp. Oregano

1 tsp. Chinese Five-Spice

<u>Directions</u>

1. Fry onions in one pan. Fill another pan with water and boil the shitake mushrooms. Lastly, get a third pan and sear off the pork hock in butter until it turns crispy.

2. Add all ingredients to your crock pot and stir well to combine and let it cook on high heat for 2 hours.

3. Stir everything together and let cook for another 2 hours on low heat. Take out the pork hock from the crock pot and de-bone it.

4. Slice as desired and return to the sauce in the crockpot. Mix thoroughly to let the pork absorb enough flavor.

5. Serve with steamed vegetables, top with vegetables.

Nutritional Information Per Serving

Calories 520, Fat 29g, Net Carbs8g & Protein 22g.

Wine & Coffee Beef Stew
Servings: 6

Ingredients

1 Cup Beef Stock

2.5 Pounds Stew Meat

3 Cups Coffee

2/3 Cup Red Wine

1 ½ Cup Mushrooms

3 tbsp. Coconut Oil

1 Medium Onion

2 tsp. Garlic

2 tbsp. Capers

1 tsp. Salt

1 tsp. Pepper

Directions

1. Cube stew meat, then slice mushrooms and onions thinly.

2. In a pan on the stove, bring coconut oil to its smoking point.

3. Season the beef with salt and pepper. In small batches to avoid overcrowding, brown all of it in the pan.

4. Once all is browned, add mushrooms, garlic and onions to the remaining fat in the pan and cook until onions are translucent.

5. Add beef stock, coffee, capers and red wine to the veggies and stir this mixture.

6. Next, add beef to the mixture, bring it to a boil, turn down heat to low and cover.

7. Cook for 3 hours and serve.

Nutritional Information Per Serving

Calories 504, Fat 32.2g, Net Carbs2.7g & Protein 42.5g.

Shrimp & Cauliflower Curry

Servings: 6

<u>Ingredients</u>

1 Cup Unsweetened Coconut Milk

4 Cups Chicken Stock

24 Oz. Shrimp

5 Cups Raw Spinach

1/2 Head Medium Cauliflower

1 Medium Onion, sliced

1/4 Cup Heavy Cream

3 tbsp. Olive Oil

1 tbsp. Coconut Flour

2 tbsp. Curry Powder

1 tbsp. Cumin

1 tsp. Chili Powder

1/4 tsp. Cinnamon

1/2 tsp. Turmeric

2 tsp. Garlic Powder

1 tsp. Onion powder

1 tsp. Paprika

1/2 tsp. Coriander

1 tsp. Cayenne

1/2 tsp. Ginger (ground, dried)

1/2 tsp. Pepper

1/4 tsp. Xanthan Gum

1/4 tsp. Cardamom

1/4 Cup Butter

Salt & Pepper to taste

Directions

1. Mix all the spices (except coconut flour and xanthan), set aside.

2. In a pan, heat olive oil over high heat. Add onion and cook onion until soft.

3. Add heavy cream, butter, spices and 1/8 tsp of xanthan, stirring them in so everything is well-mixed.

4. After 1-2 minutes, add chicken broth and coconut milk. Stir thoroughly and cover.

5. Cook for 30 minutes. Chop the cauliflower into small florets then add it to curry. Cook for 15 minutes more still covered.

6. Detail shrimp and devein, then add to the curry. Cook additional 1 to20 minutes, uncovered.

7. Measure out coconut flour and 1/8 tsp. xanthan gum and stir well into curry. Let it cook for 5 minutes.

8. Now add spinach and mix well. Cook for 5 to10 minutes more with the lid off.

Nutritional Information Per Serving

Calories 331, Fat 19.5g, Net Carbs5.6.g & Protein 27.4g.

Cabbage Rolls & Corned Beef
Servings: 5

<u>Ingredients</u>

3.5 lbs. Corned Beef

1 Medium Onion

1 tsp. Whole Peppercorns

15 Savoy Cabbage Leaves

1 Fresh Lemon

1 tbsp. Brown Mustard

1/4 Cup White Wine

1/4 Cup Coffee

1 tsp. Mustard Seeds

1 tbsp. Bacon Fat

2 tsp. Kosher Salt

1 Crushed Bay Leaf

1 tbsp. Erythritol

2 tsp. Worcestershire

1/4 tsp. Cloves

1/2 tsp. Red Pepper Flakes

1/4 tsp. Allspice

<u>Directions</u>

1. Add your liquids, corned beef and spices to crockpot and let it cook on low for 6 hours.

2. Next, boil a pot of water. Add all the cabbage leaves and 1 Sliced Onion to the boiling water and leave for 2 to3 minutes.

3. Remove cabbage from water and blanch in ice water for 3 to 4 minutes. Keep boiling the onion in the water.

4. Dry off cabbage leaves, slice meat, add onions and then roll the fillings into the cabbage leaves.

Nutritional Information Per Serving

Calories 478, Fats25g, Net Carbs3.8g, Protein 34.2g

Szechuan Keto Chicken

Ingredients

1 1/2 lbs. Ground Chicken

1/2 Cup Chicken Stock

6 Cups Spinach

4 Tbsp. Organic Tomato Paste

2 Tbsp. Chili Garlic Paste

3 Tbsp. Coconut Oil

1/2 tsp. Minced Ginger

2 Tbsp. Soy Sauce

1 Tbsp. Red Wine Vinegar

1 tsp. Red Pepper Flakes

1 Tbsp. + 1 tsp. Erythritol

2 tsp. Spicy Brown Mustard

2 tsp. Salt

2 tsp. Pepper

1/2 tsp. Mrs. Dash Table Blend

Directions

1. In a ramekin, mix soy sauce, tomato paste, brown mustard, chili garlic paste and ginger together.

2. Bring coconut oil to medium-high heat. Season ground chicken with salt and pepper, cook in the oil until cooked through. Break into small pieces.

3. Add 2/3 of sauce to the mixture, mixing well. Add spinach to chicken and leave to wilt. Add red pepper flakes, Mrs. Dash seasoning, salt and pepper.

4. Add the last 1/3 sauce, red wine vinegar, chicken stock and erythritol. Stir the spices and spinach in well.

5. Reduce heat to low, cover pan and cook for 10-15 minutes.

Nutritional Information Per Serving

Calories 387, Fats28.8g, Net Carbs3.9g, Protein 47.3g

Chili Dinner Pot

Servings: 4

<u>Ingredients</u>

2 Tbsp. Soy Sauce

2 lbs. Stew Meat

1/3 Cup Tomato Paste

1 Medium Onion

1 Cup Beef Broth

1 Medium Green Pepper

2 Tbsp. Olive Oil

1 1/2 tsp. Cumin

2 Tbsp. + 1 tsp. Chili Powder

2 tsp. Red Boat Fish Sauce

2 tsp. Paprika

2 tsp. Minced Garlic

1 tsp. Oregano

1 tsp. Worcestershire

1 tsp. Cayenne Pepper

1 tsp. Black Pepper

1 tsp. Salt

Optional: for a more watery chili, add 1 Cup Coffee.

<u>Direction</u>

1. Cube half of the stew meat into small cubes. In a food processor, process the other half into the ground beef.

2. Chop onion and pepper into small pieces. Mix together all spices to make sauce.

3. In a pan, sauté cubed beef until browned and transfer to a crockpot. Treat the ground beef the same way.

4. Sauté the veggies in the remaining fat that is in the pan until the onions are translucent.

5. Add them all to the crockpot and mix together.

6. Finally, simmer on high for 2 1/2 hours. Simmer again for 20 to 30 minutes uncovered.

<u>Nutritional Information Per Serving</u>

Calories 398, Fats 17.8g, Net Carbs5.3g, Protein 51.8g

Pork Loin Ribs With Barbecue Sauce

Serving: 4

<u>Ingredients</u>

For the Pork Loin Ribs:

1 1/2 Cups of Char-Broil Mesquite Smoking Chips

3 Racks (8.15 lbs) Pork Loin Back Ribs

3 Tbsp. Liquid Smoke

1 Tbsp of Southwest Seasoning

3 Tbsp. Salt

3 Tbsp. Pepper

1 Tbsp. Garlic Powder

For the Keto BBQ Sauce:

1/2 tsp. Cumin

2 tsp. Yellow Mustard

1/2 Cup Ketchup, Sugar -Free

1 tsp. Liquid Smoke

1 Tbsp. Hot Sauce

1 tsp. Worcestershire

1/2 tsp. Chili Powder

1/4 tsp. Cayenne Pepper

1/2 tsp. of Mrs. Dash Table Blend

Direction

1. Preheat the oven to 225F. Dig fingers through the centre of ribs and pull it back to remove the silverskin from the ribs.

2. Season sides of ribs with a generous amount of salt and pepper.

3. Add the garlic powder and liquid smoke then rub it all into the ribs.

4. Cover baking pan with foil and place into the oven for 2 hours. Increase oven to 250F and keep cooking for 2 hours more.

5. Add together the sauce ingredients and mix well. Allow the ribs to rest for about 10 minutes then transfer to foil.

6. Soak the wood chips, brush the ribs with the sauce and smoke it on medium high heat for 60-90 minutes.

7. Finish off the ribs on the grill for 10-12 minutes per side.

8. Spread remaining sauce as you serve.

Nutritional Information Per Serving

Calories 785, Fats 62.1g, Net Carbs1.5g, Protein 56g

Perfect Family Roast

Yields: 8

<u>Ingredients</u>

1 tsp. Garlic Powder

5 lbs. Beef Rib Roast

2 tsp. Salt

1 tsp. Pepper

<u>Directions:</u>

1. Let the roast attain room temperature for 1 full hour.

2. Next, Preheat oven to 375F then mix together all the spices.

3. Place roast inside a casserole dish or onto a roasting rack and rub with spices.

4. Roast in the oven for 1 hour. Turn oven off completely. Do not open the door but let the roast sit in the oven for 3 hours.

5. 30 to 45 minutes before serving, turn the oven back on to 375F.

6. Take out roast from oven and leave to rest for about 10 minutes then cut and serving.

<u>Nutritional Information Per Serving</u>

Calories 681, Fats 46.6g, Net Carbs0.3g, Protein 90g

Sunset Cuban

Serving: 1

<u>Ingredients</u>

37g Raw ground beef

14g butter

11g raw onion, thinly diced

25g canned tomato in puree or juice

15g green olives, thinly sliced

Salt/pepper, garlic powder, red pepper flakes , oregano ground cumin (all optional)

10g coconut oil (serve on the side)

<u>Directions</u>

1. Sauté butter and ground beef in a small skillet over medium heat. Don't drain the fat!

2. Add the onions and cook until it is translucent.

3. Add the green olives, tomato puree and desired seasonings. Add a little water to make it simmer longer.

4. Let the mixture simmer until flavors are thoroughly combined.

5. Add the remaining fat and serve.

<u>Nutritional Information Per Serving</u>

Calories 300, Net Carbs2.19g, Protein 7.48g